# 10 BENEFITS OF
## GOING GLUTEN-FREE

- Improves cholesterol levels
- Promotes digestive health
- Increases energy levels
- Eliminates unhealthy and processed foods from your diet (oils, fried food, breads, and desserts to name a few)
- More likely to eat fruits and vegetables because they are all gluten-free
- Reduces your risk of heart disease, certain cancers, and diabetes
- Helps ward off viruses and germs as many foods you will now eat will contain more antioxidants, vitamins, and minerals
- Promotes healthy weight-loss
- Improves health of people with irritable bowl syndrome and arthritis
- Distinctly improved awareness of foods that can have an adverse effect on your health

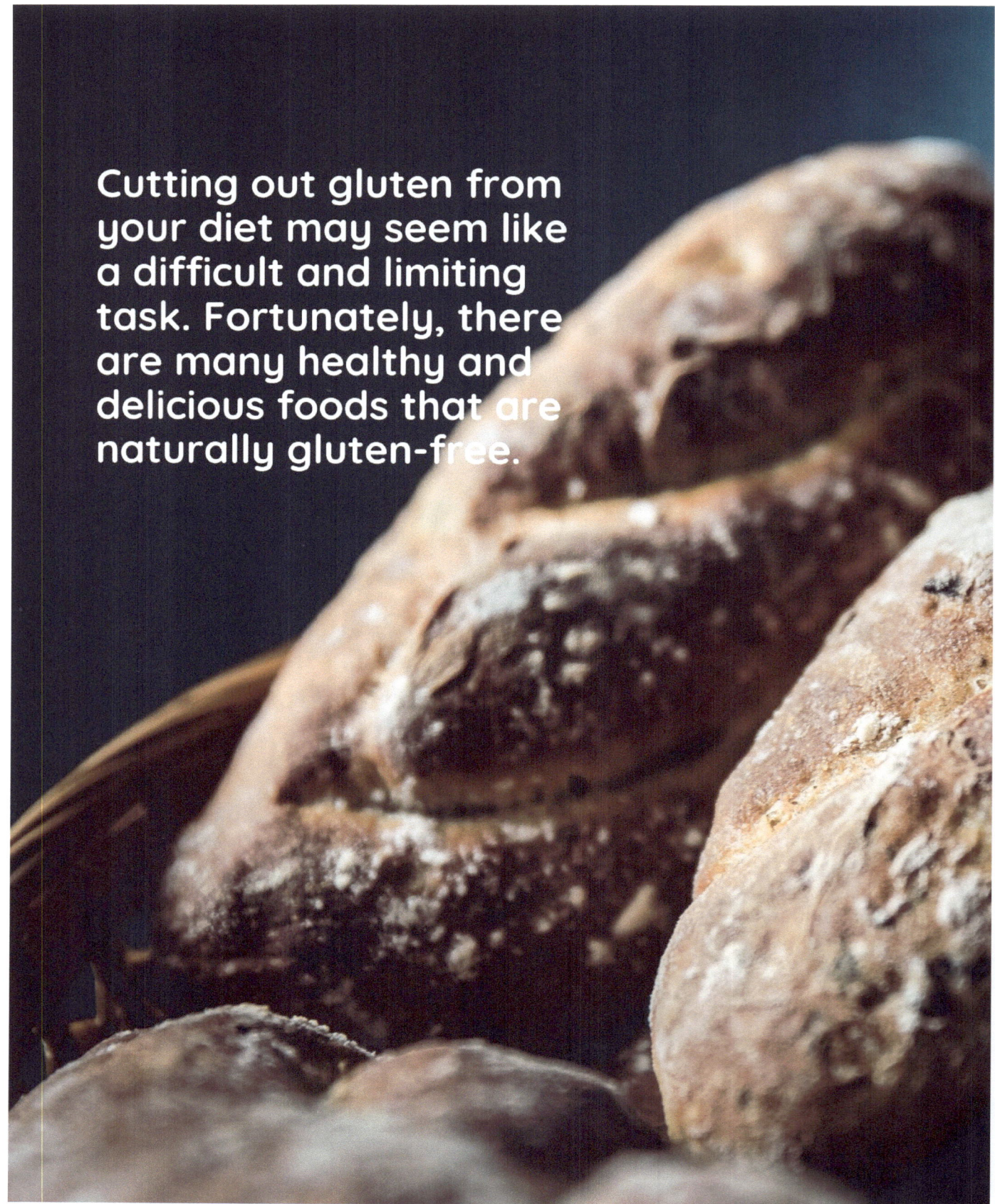

Cutting out gluten from your diet may seem like a difficult and limiting task. Fortunately, there are many healthy and delicious foods that are naturally gluten-free.

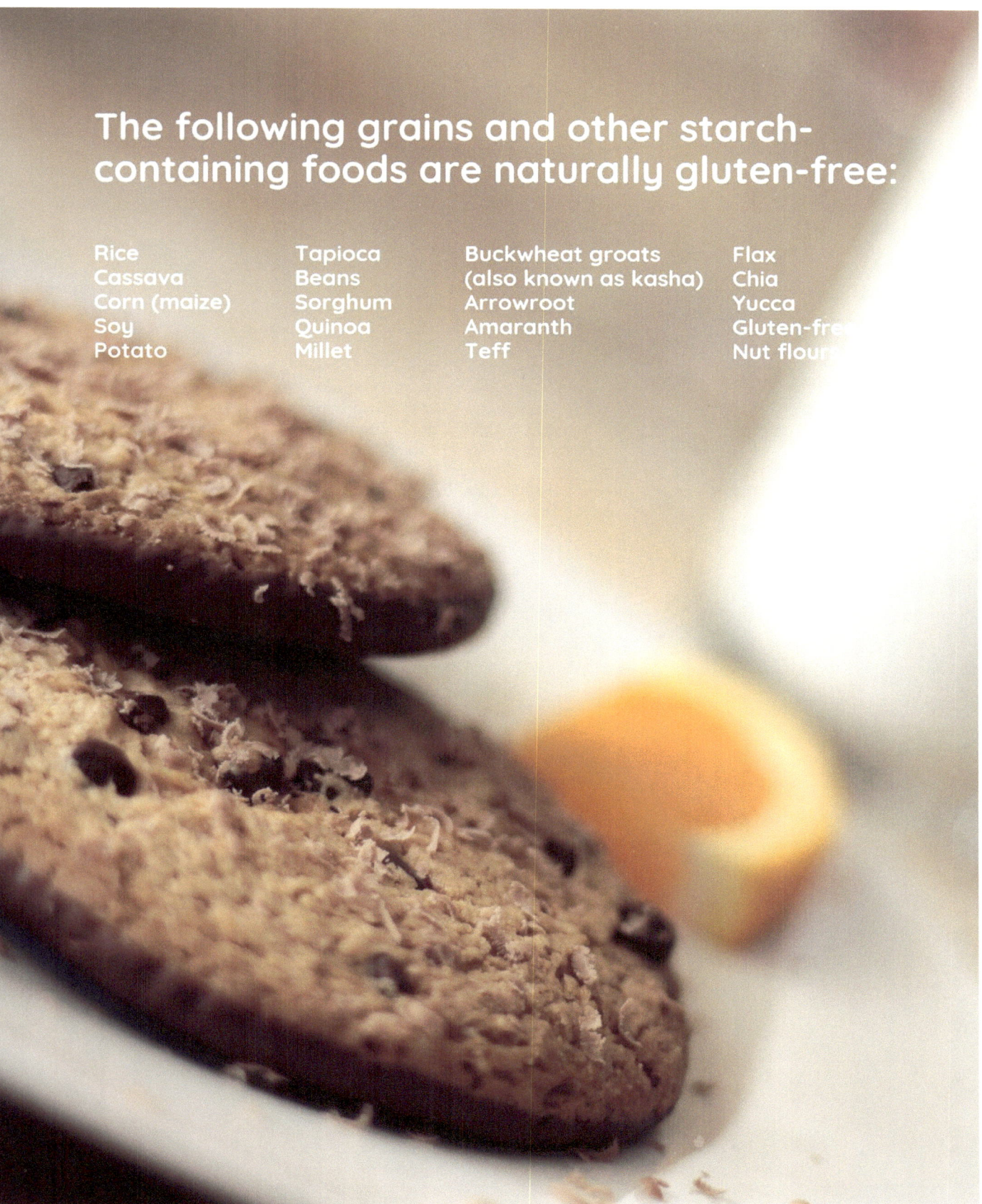

# The following grains and other starch-containing foods are naturally gluten-free:

| | | | |
|---|---|---|---|
| Rice | Tapioca | Buckwheat groats | Flax |
| Cassava | Beans | (also known as kasha) | Chia |
| Corn (maize) | Sorghum | Arrowroot | Yucca |
| Soy | Quinoa | Amaranth | Gluten-free |
| Potato | Millet | Teff | Nut flours |

# Gluten-Free Thai Chicken Soup

## Ingredients

1 tablespoon grapeseed oil
3 shallots, chopped
2 tablespoons chopped cilantro
4 cups chicken stock
2 (14 ounce) cans coconut milk
1 tablespoon agave nectar
1 (8 ounce) package crimini mushrooms, sliced
1 head broccoli, cut into florets
1 pound thinly sliced chicken breast meat
2 teaspoons red curry paste
3 tablespoons lime juice
3 tablespoons fish sauce

1/2 cup chopped fresh cilantro
2 serrano chile peppers, thinly sliced
1/4 cup chopped green onions
8 lime wedges

## Directions

Heat the grapeseed oil in a large saucepan over medium heat. Cook and stir the shallots and 2 tablespoons chopped cilantro in the hot pan until the shallot has softened and turned translucent, about 4 minutes. Pour in the chicken stock, coconut milk, and agave nectar; bring to a simmer over medium-high heat. Once the broth reaches a simmer, strain through a mesh strainer into a clean saucepan; discard the shallot and cilantro.

Return the broth to a simmer; stir in the mushrooms and broccoli and cook until the broccoli becomes tender, about 4 minutes. Add the chicken and cook until no longer pink, stirring constantly. Stir the curry paste, lime juice, and fish sauce in a small bowl to dissolve the curry paste; mix into the simmering soup.

Ladle the soup into bowls and sprinkle with 1/2 cup cilantro, serrano peppers, green onions, and lime wedges to serve.

# Gluten-Free Golden Yam Brownies

## Ingredients

2 tablespoons dry egg replacer (such as Ener-G®)
1/2 cup water
1 1/2 cups sweet rice flour (mochiko)
1 1/2 teaspoons xanthan gum
1 teaspoon baking powder
1/2 teaspoon salt
1 cup vegan margarine (such as Earth Balance®)
1 cup packed brown sugar
1 cup turbinado sugar (such as Sugar in the Raw®)
2 teaspoons gluten-free vanilla extract
2 cups peeled and finely shredded yam

3/4 cup turbinado sugar (such as Sugar in the Raw®)
1/4 cup cornstarch
2 tablespoons vegan margarine (such as Earth Balance®), softened
2 tablespoons almond milk

## Directions

Preheat an oven to 350 degrees F (175 degrees C). Grease a 9x13-inch baking dish.

Stir the egg replacer and water together in a small bowl until the powder is completely integrated. Stir the rice flour, xanthan gum, baking powder, and salt together in a separate bowl.

Beat 1 cup margarine, brown sugar, and 1 cup turbinado sugar with an electric mixer in a large bowl until light and fluffy. Add the egg replacer about 1/2 cup at a time, allowing each addition to blend into the butter mixture before adding the next. Add the vanilla extract with the last of the egg replacer. Pour the rice flour mixture into the batter, mixing until just incorporated. Fold the shredded yam into the batter, mixing just enough to evenly combine. Pour the batter into prepared pan.

Bake in the preheated oven until a toothpick inserted into the center comes out clean, about 30 minutes.

Stir 3/4 cup turbinado sugar, cornstarch, 2 tablespoons margarine, and almond milk together in a small bowl until smooth. Spread over the brownies while still warm; they will absorb some of the glaze. Serve warm.

# Gluten-Free Yellow Cake

## Ingredients

1 1/2 cups white rice flour
3/4 cup tapioca flour
1 teaspoon salt
1 teaspoon baking soda
3 teaspoons baking powder
1 teaspoon xanthan gum
4 eggs
1 1/4 cups white sugar
2/3 cup mayonnaise
1 cup milk
2 teaspoons gluten-free vanilla extract

## Directions

Preheat oven to 350 degrees F (175 degrees C). Grease and rice flour two 8 or 9 inch round cake pans.

Mix the white rice flour, tapioca flour, salt, baking soda, baking powder and xanthan gum together and set aside.

Mix the eggs, sugar, and mayonnaise until fluffy. Add the flour mixture, milk and vanilla and mix well. Spread batter into the prepared pans.

Bake at 350 degrees F (175 degrees C) for 25 minutes. Cakes are done when they spring back when lightly touched or when a toothpick inserted near the center comes out clean. Let cool completely then frost, if desired.

# Perfect Gluten-Free Peanut Butter Cookies

## Ingredients

1/2 cup gluten free, casein free margarine
1/2 cup brown sugar
1/2 cup white sugar
1 egg
1/2 cup salted natural peanut butter
1/2 teaspoon baking soda
1 cup soy flour
1/4 cup tapioca flour
1/4 cup potato flour

## Directions

Preheat the oven to 375 degrees F (190 degrees C).

In a medium bowl, cream together the margarine, brown sugar and white sugar until smooth. Mix in the egg and peanut butter. Combine the baking soda, soy flour, tapioca flour and potato flour; stir into the batter to form a dough. Roll teaspoonfuls of dough into balls and place them 2 inches apart onto ungreased baking sheets.

Bake for 8 to 10 minutes in the preheated oven. Allow cookies to cool on baking sheet for 5 minutes before removing to a wire rack to cool completely.

# Gluten-Free Irish Soda Bread

## Ingredients

1 1/2 cups white rice flour
1/2 cup tapioca flour
1/2 cup white sugar
1 teaspoon baking soda
1 teaspoon baking powder
1 teaspoon salt
1 egg
1 cup buttermilk

## Directions

Preheat oven to 350 degrees F (175 degrees C).  Grease a 9 inch round cake pan.

Combine the rice flour, tapioca flour, sugar, baking soda, baking powder, and salt in a large bowl.  In a separate bowl, whisk together egg and buttermilk . Make a well in the center of the dry ingredients and pour in the wet. Stir just until the dry ingredients are moistened. Pour into the cake pan.

Bake for 65 minutes in the preheated oven, or until a toothpick inserted into the center comes out clean.  Cool on a wire rack, for 10 minutes before removing from the pan.  Wrap bread in plastic wrap or aluminum foil and let stand overnight for the best flavor.

# Delicious Gluten-Free Pancakes

## Ingredients

1 cup rice flour
3 tablespoons tapioca flour
1/3 cup potato starch
4 tablespoons dry buttermilk powder
1 packet sugar substitute
1 1/2 teaspoons baking powder
1/2 teaspoon baking soda
1/2 teaspoon salt
1/2 teaspoon xanthan gum
2 eggs
3 tablespoons canola oil
2 cups water

## Directions

In a bowl, mix or sift together the rice flour, tapioca flour, potato starch, dry buttermilk powder, sugar substitute, baking powder, baking soda, salt, and xanthan gum. Stir in eggs, water, and oil until well blended and few lumps remain.

Heat a large, well-oiled skillet or griddle over medium high heat. Spoon batter onto skillet and cook until bubbles begin to form. Flip, and continue cooking until golden brown on bottom. Serve immediately with condiments of your choice.

# Gluten-Free Chocolate Cake with Semi-Sweet

## Ingredients

1/2 cup sorghum flour
1/2 cup tapioca flour
1/2 cup rice flour
1 cup cocoa powder, sifted
1 1/2 tablespoons xanthan gum
2 1/2 teaspoons baking powder
1 teaspoon baking soda
3/4 cup butter at room temperature
3/4 cup (packed) dark brown sugar
1 cup white sugar
3 eggs
2 egg yolks
2 teaspoons vanilla extract
1 1/2 cups buttermilk

5 ounces chocolate chips
1/2 cup sour cream
1/2 teaspoon vanilla extract
1 tablespoon heavy cream

## Directions

Preheat oven to 350 degrees F (175 degrees C). Grease a 9x13 inch pan and set aside.

In a medium bowl, sift together the sorghum, tapioca, and rice flours with the cocoa powder, xanthan gum, baking powder, and baking soda.

In a large mixer bowl, cream the butter until light and fluffy. Slowly beat in the brown and white sugars; whip until fluffy. Beat in the eggs and egg yolks one at a time. Add the vanilla. On low speed, alternately combine the buttermilk with the flour mixture. Pour batter into prepared pan.

Bake in preheated oven for 30 to 35 minutes, or until a toothpick inserted into the center of the cake comes out clean. Cool in pan.

To make the icing, in the top of a double boiler over medium high heat, melt the chocolate chips (or use microwave). Remove from heat and cool until warm. Stir in the sour cream and vanilla; add heavy cream. Stir in additional heavy cream to make desired consistency. Once the cake is thoroughly cool, spread a thin layer of frosting over the top.

# Amazing Gluten-free Layer Bars

## Ingredients

7 ounces flaked coconut
1 cup butterscotch chips
6 ounces semisweet chocolate chips
8 ounces unsalted peanuts
1/2 cup sliced almonds
1 (14 ounce) can sweetened condensed milk

## Directions

Preheat oven to 350 degrees F ( 175 degrees C ). Generously grease one 13x9 inch baking pan.

Spread 2/3 of the flaked coconut evenly on the bottom of the baking pan. Sprinkle the butterscotch morsel, chocolate chips, and peanuts evenly over the coconut layer. Pour condensed milk evenly over the whole pan. Top with sliced almonds and remaining coconut . Bake for 20 minutes in the preheated oven. Cool completely before cutting into squares.

# Gluten Free Macadamia Pie Crust

## Ingredients

6 ounces macadamia nuts
2 eggs
1 1/2 cups soy flour

## Directions

Preheat the oven to 350 degrees F (175 degrees C).

Place the macadamia nuts into the container of a food processor, and blend until they reach a peanut butter like consistency. Scrape out into a bowl, and stir in the eggs and soy flour until well blended.

Place the dough between two pieces of waxed paper, and roll out into about a 12 inch circle. Remove the top piece of waxed paper, and invert the dough into a 9 inch pie plate. Press into the bottom and up the sides. Remove any overhanging dough.

Bake for 5 minutes in the preheated oven, or until light golden brown. Use in any recipe calling for a prebaked pie crust.

# Perfect Cashew and Peanut Butter Gluten-free

## Ingredients

1/2 cup brown sugar
1/2 cup white sugar
1 egg
1/4 cup salted natural peanut butter
1/4 cup cashew butter
1/2 cup gluten free, casein free margarine
1/2 teaspoon baking soda
1/2 cup corn flour
1/2 cup tapioca flour
1/4 cup potato flour

## Directions

Preheat oven to 350 degrees F (175 degrees C).

In a medium bowl, mix together the margarine, brown sugar, white sugar and egg until smooth. Stir in the peanut butter and cashew butter. Combine the baking soda, corn flour, tapioca flour, and potato flour; stir into the batter to form a dough. Roll the dough into teaspoon sized balls and place them 2 inches apart onto an ungreased cookie sheet.

Bake for 8 to 10 minutes in the preheated oven. Let cool on baking sheets for a few minutes before removing to wire racks to cool completely.

# Gluten Free Chocolate Cupcakes

## Ingredients

1 1/2 cups white rice flour
3/4 cup millet flour
1/2 cup unsweetened cocoa powder
1 teaspoon salt
1 teaspoon baking soda
1 tablespoon baking powder
1 teaspoon xanthan gum
4 eggs
1 1/4 cups white sugar
2/3 cup sour cream
1 cup milk
2 teaspoons vanilla extract

## Directions

Preheat oven to 350 degrees F (175 degrees C). Grease two 12 cup muffin pans or line with paper baking cups.

In a medium bowl, stir together the rice flour, millet flour, cocoa, salt, baking soda, baking powder and xanathan gum. In a separate large bowl, beat the eggs, sugar, sour cream, milk and vanilla. Stir in the dry ingredients until smooth. Spoon the batter into the prepared cups, dividing evenly.

Bake in the preheated oven until the tops spring back when lightly pressed, 20 to 25 minutes. Cool in the pan set over a wire rack. When cool, arrange the cupcakes on a serving platter.

# Garbanzo Bean Chocolate Cake (Gluten Free!)

## Ingredients

1 1/2 cups semisweet chocolate chips
1 (19 ounce) can garbanzo beans, rinsed and drained
4 eggs
3/4 cup white sugar
1/2 teaspoon baking powder
1 tablespoon confectioners' sugar for dusting

## Directions

Preheat the oven to 350 degrees F (175 degrees C). Grease and flour a 9 inch round cake pan.

Place the chocolate chips into a microwave-safe bowl. Cook in the microwave for about 2 minutes, stirring every 20 seconds after the first minute, until chocolate is melted and smooth. If you have a powerful microwave, reduce the power to 50 percent.

Combine the beans and eggs in the bowl of a food processor. Process until smooth. Add the sugar and the baking powder, and pulse to blend. Pour in the melted chocolate and blend until smooth, scraping down the corners to make sure chocolate is completely mixed. Transfer the batter to the prepared cake pan.

Bake for 40 minutes in the preheated oven, or until a knife inserted into the center of the cake comes out clean. Cool in the pan on a wire rack for 10 to 15 minutes before inverting onto a serving plate. Dust with confectioners' sugar just before serving.

# Golly Gee Gluten-Free Pancakes

## Ingredients

1 egg
1/4 cup apple juice
1 tablespoon unsalted butter,
melted
1/4 cup amaranth flour
1/4 cup tapioca flour
3 tablespoons arrowroot flour
1/4 teaspoon ground cinnamon
1 pinch ground nutmeg
1/2 teaspoon wheat-free baking
powder
1/4 teaspoon salt

## Directions

In a medium mixing bowl, beat the egg with the apple juice and melted butter. Add the remaining ingredients and stir.

Heat a lightly oiled griddle or frying pan over medium high heat. Pour or scoop the batter onto the griddle, using approximately 1/4 cup for each pancake. Brown on both sides and serve hot. This batter must be used right away and can not sit and wait.

# Gluten-free Peanut Butter Cookies

## Ingredients

2 cups peanut butter
2 cups white sugar
4 eggs, beaten
2 cups semi-sweet chocolate chips (optional)
1 1/2 cups chopped pecans (optional)

## Directions

Preheat oven to 350 degrees F (175 degrees C). Grease cookie sheet.

Combine peanut butter, eggs, and sugar and mix until smooth. Mix in chocolate chips and nuts, if desired. Spoon dough by tablespoons onto a cookie sheet.

Bake for 10 to 12 minutes or until lightly browned. Let the cookies cool on the cookie sheets for 5 to 10 minutes before removing.

# Gluten-free Mexican Wedding Cakes

## Ingredients

1/2 cup butter
1 teaspoon gluten free vanilla extract
1 cup confectioners' sugar
1/2 cup white rice flour
1/4 cup cornstarch
1/4 cup tapioca flour
1/4 teaspoon unflavored gelatin (optional)
1 cup chopped hazelnuts
1 cup chopped walnuts or hazelnuts
confectioners' sugar for dusting

## Directions

Preheat the oven to 350 degrees F (175 degrees C).

In a medium bowl, mix together the butter and vanilla until well blended. Sift together the confectioners' sugar, rice flour, cornstarch, tapioca starch and gelatin. Stir into the butter mixture until all of the dry ingredients have been absorbed. Mix in the ground hazelnuts and chopped hazelnuts. Form teaspoonfuls of dough into balls, and shape into crescents. Place cookies at least 2 inches apart onto ungreased cookie sheets.

Bake for 8 to 10 minutes in the preheated oven, until golden brown. For crispier cookies, reduce heat to 325 degrees F (165 degrees C), and bake slightly longer. When cookies have cooled completely, dust with additional confectioners' sugar.

# Alison's Gluten Free Bread

## Ingredients

1 egg
1/3 cup egg whites
1 tablespoon apple cider vinegar
1/4 cup canola oil
1/4 cup honey
1 1/2 cups warm skim milk
1 teaspoon salt
1 tablespoon xanthan gum
1/2 cup tapioca flour
1/4 cup garbanzo bean flour
1/4 cup millet flour
1 cup white rice flour
1 cup brown rice flour
1 tablespoon active dry yeast

## Directions

Place ingredients in the pan of the bread machine in the order recommended by the manufacturer. Select cycle; press Start. Five minutes into the cycle, check the consistency of the dough. Add additional rice flour or liquid if necessary.

When bread is finished, let cool for 10 to 15 minutes before removing from pan.

# Gluten-Free Pie Crust with LIBBY'S® Famous

## Ingredients

Crust:
1 cup white rice flour
1/2 cup potato starch
1/2 cup tapioca flour
1/4 teaspoon salt
6 tablespoons cold butter, cut into small pieces
1 large egg, beaten
1 tablespoon apple cider or white vinegar
3 tablespoons ice water, or as needed

Filling:
1 1/2 cups granulated sugar
1 teaspoon salt
2 teaspoons ground cinnamon
1 teaspoon ground ginger
1/2 teaspoon ground cloves
4 large eggs
1 (29 ounce) can LIBBY'S® 100% Pure Pumpkin
2 (12 fluid ounce) cans NESTLE® CARNATION® Evaporated Milk
Whipped cream or topping (optional)

## Directions

For Pie Crust: Combine rice flour, potato starch, tapioca flour and salt in medium bowl. Cut in butter with pastry blender or two knives until mixture is crumbly. Form well in center. Add egg and vinegar; stir gently with a fork until just blended. Sprinkle with water; blend together with a fork and clean hands until mixture just holds together and forms a ball. (Be careful not to add too much water as dough will be hard to roll.)

Shape dough into ball and divide in half. Cover one half with plastic wrap; set aside. Place remaining half on lightly floured (use rice flour) sheet of wax paper. Top with additional piece of wax paper. Roll out dough to 1/8-inch thickness. Remove top sheet of wax paper and invert dough into 9-inch deep-dish (4-cup volume) pie plate. Slowly peel away wax paper. Trim excess crust. Turn edge under; crimp as desired. Repeat with remaining half.

For Filling: Mix sugar, salt, cinnamon, ginger and cloves in small bowl. Beat eggs in large bowl. Stir in pumpkin and sugar-spice mixture. Gradually stir in evaporated milk. POUR into pie shells.

Bake in preheated 425 degrees F. oven for 15 minutes. Reduce temperature to 350 degrees F.; bake for 40 to 50 minutes or until knife inserted near center comes out clean. Cool on wire rack for 2 hours. Serve immediately or refrigerate. Top with whipped cream or topping before serving.

# Chocolate Chip Cookies (Gluten Free)

## Ingredients

3/4 cup butter, softened
1 1/4 cups packed brown sugar
1/4 cup white sugar
1 teaspoon gluten-free vanilla extract
1/4 cup egg substitute
2 1/4 cups gluten-free baking mix
1 teaspoon baking soda
1 teaspoon baking powder
1 teaspoon salt
12 ounces semisweet chocolate chips

## Directions

Preheat oven to 375 degrees F ( 190 degrees C). Prepare a greased baking sheet.

In a medium bowl, cream butter and sugar. Gradually add replacer eggs and vanilla while mixing. Sift together gluten- free flour mix, baking soda, baking powder, and salt. Stir into the butter mixture until blended. Finally, stir in the chocolate chips.

Using a  teaspoon, drop cookies 2 inches apart on prepared baking sheet. Bake in preheated oven for 6 to 8 minutes or until light brown. Let cookies cool on baking sheet for 2 minutes before removing to wire racks.

# Gluten-Free Fudge Brownies

## Ingredients

2/3 cup gluten-free baking mix (such as Bob's Red Mill All Purpose GF Baking Flour®)
1/2 cup cornstarch
1 cup white sugar
1 cup packed brown sugar
3/4 cup unsweetened cocoa powder
1 teaspoon baking soda
2 eggs, beaten
3/4 cup margarine, melted

## Directions

Preheat oven to 350 degrees F (175 degrees C), and grease an 8x8 inch square baking dish.

Stir together the gluten-free baking mix, cornstarch, white sugar, brown sugar, cocoa powder, and baking soda in a bowl, sifting with a fork to remove lumps.  Pour in the eggs and melted margarine, and mix with a large spoon or electric mixer on low until the mixture forms a smooth batter, 3 to 5 minutes. Scrape the batter into the prepared baking dish.

Place a sheet of aluminum foil on the oven rack to prevent spills as the brownies rise, then fall during baking. Bake until a toothpick inserted in the center of the brownies comes out clean, 40 to 45 minutes.

# Gluten-Free Orange Almond Cake with Orange

## Ingredients

3 eggs, separated
2/3 cup white sugar
1/4 cup rice flour
1 teaspoon ground cinnamon
1/2 cup orange juice
1 1/2 cups finely ground almonds
(almond meal)

2 tablespoons heavy cream
2 cups white sugar
1 cup orange juice
1 tablespoon grated orange zest
1/2 cup butter
4 egg whites

## Directions

Preheat the oven to 325 degrees F (165 degrees C). Grease a 10 inch springform pan with cooking spray, and dust with rice flour.

In a large bowl, whip egg yolks with 2/3 cup of sugar until thick and pale using an electric mixer. This will take about 5 minutes. Stir in the rice flour and orange juice, then fold in the almond meal and cinnamon.

In a separate glass or metal bowl, whip 3 egg whites until they can hold a stiff peak. Fold into the almond mixture until well blended. Pour into the prepared pan, and spread evenly.

Bake for 35 to 40 minutes in the preheated oven, until a toothpick inserted into the center comes out clean. Cool in the pan on a wire rack. Run a knife around the outer edge of the cake to help remove it from the pan.

To make the orange sauce, cream together the butter and 2 cups of white sugar in a medium bowl. Stir in the cream, and place the dish over a pan of barely simmering water. Stir in orange juice and zest. Whip 4 egg whites in a separate bowl until soft peaks form. Fold into the orange sauce. Spoon over the cake and serve immediately.

# Dairy and Gluten-Free 'Buttermilk Pancakes'

## Ingredients

1 cup sweet rice flour
2 teaspoons baking powder
1/2 teaspoon baking soda
1/2 teaspoon ground cinnamon
(optional)
1/2 teaspoon salt
2 eggs, beaten
1 1/4 cups soy yogurt
1/4 cup rice milk
2 tablespoons vegetable oil

## Directions

Sift the rice flour, baking powder, baking soda, cinnamon, and salt
in a bowl. In another bowl, whisk together the beaten eggs, soy
yogurt, rice milk, and oil, and pour into the flour mixture. Stir briefly
just to combine.

Heat a lightly oiled griddle or frying pan over medium-high heat.
Scoop about 1/4 cup of batter per pancake onto the heated griddle,
and cook for 1 to 2 minutes, until bubbles appear on the surface.
Flip the pancake and cook 1 to 2 minutes more, until the pancake is
golden brown on both sides.